UNLIKELY DANCER WORKBOOK

DEBBIE MALONE

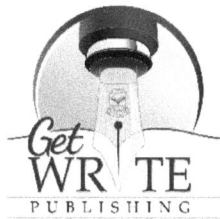

Get
WRITE
PUBLISHING

ISBN: 978-1-945456-48-0 (Paperback)

Any references to historical events, real people, or real places are used fictitiously. Names, characters, and places are products of the author's imagination.

The events in the book are the author's memories from *her* perspective. Certain names have been changed to protect the identities of those involved.

Book design by Warrior Design Company.

First printing edition 2019.

www.inclusioneducation.com

Table of Contents

Introduction

The first two books in this *Unlikely Dancer* series bring us to the point of applying the knowledge and commitment of full inclusion of people with disabilities in the life of the church.

We began with a memoir about disability, tragedy, and healing. We experienced the traumatic auto accident that disrupted a happy, productive, and fulfilled life. We joined the rehabilitation process through the eyes of a person who already had a disability.

In *Unlikely Dancer 2* we used the author's experiences to demonstrate the problems and solutions associated with including individuals and families affected by disability. We discussed conceptual and practical ideas that can be used in many types of organizations that wish to be inclusive of people with disabilities.

In this *Unlikely Dancer Workbook*, we delve into the practical steps that will propel your organization forward. At the conclusion of this journey we will know where we stand, where we want to go, and the steps it will take to get there. We will evaluate the current status of our church and develop a plan of action toward a fully functioning body that appreciates and utilizes all the gifts and talents of the people. We will work alongside each other for the advancement of the Kingdom of God.

Oftentimes, disability ministry is started by one or two people with a heart for change. Before beginning any evaluations or suggestions, get permissions from your pastor and leaders. Explain your heart for people with disabilities. Involve them in the process.

Start building your team right from the start. As you go through the process you will find people who are committed to people with disabilities. Ask them to be part of the ministry. Allow others to help you. Each person has a unique viewpoint and purpose. Build the disability ministry team as soon as possible in the process.

The process will involve personal growth. You will look inside yourself, discover your attitudes, and experience change. Be honest with yourself. You will be brought to a new level in your knowledge and commitment.

Unlikely Dancer 2 and this *Unlikely Dancer Workbook* are divided into three phases. The Get Us phase involves the basics of providing a welcoming environment. The Keep Us phase provides conceptual and practical ideas to encourage people with disabilities to become increasingly involved in the church culture. The Use Us phase puts people with and without disabilities working and growing together.

Although these phases separate different activities and goals, they are not meant to be conducted separately. From a practical standpoint you will be working on parts of each phase at the same time. You and your church will continually be learning, growing, and practicing different concepts.

As with any type of ministry we must be respectful of people's privacy. Be careful about talking specifics concerning an individual or family affected by disability. It is wrong to inform anyone about the individual's disability or whether he/she has a disability without permission. Use generalizations in your conversations, assessments, and solutions.

As you move through the workbook you may need clarification or more viewpoints. Additional resources for each chapter are available in *Unlikely Dancer 2: 3 Phases of Disability Inclusion.*

All scriptures in this workbook are from the New International Version (NIV) unless otherwise specified.

One final word as we embark on this journey together. Pray. Pray. Pray.

Part I: Get Us

Welcome

Therefore welcome one another as Christ has welcomed you, for the glory of God.

Romans 15:7 (ESV)

Read the story of Mephibosheth in 2 Samuel 9. Describe his story in your own words. What significance does it have with welcoming people with disabilities in the church?

_____

_____

_____

_____

1.: Biblical Foundations

For you created my inmost being; you knit me together in my mother's womb. I praise you because I am fearfully and wonderfully made; your works are wonderful; I know that full well.

Ps 139:13-14

Read John 9:1-7. Why was this man born blind? What was his purpose? How did his purpose manifest itself? Did he have purpose after his healing? What was the purpose?

_____

_____

_____

_____

_____

Watch the video of Nick Vujicic - God will not give up on u..

https://www.youtube.com/watch?v=KJ1OEi2OhSU

Write your impression of Nick as a person, an evangelist, a motivator.

How is God using Nick's disability for His glory?

_____

_____

_____

_____

_____

_____

_____

_____

_____

_____

_____

Visit two churches (not your own). Observe people with disabilities.

Can you observe any people with disabilities serving in ministry? In leadership? Are there wheelchair users in the isle or all lined along the back? Are people with disabilities being segregated? Notate your observations.

_____

_____

_____

_____

_____

_____

_____

_____

_____

_____

_____

Now evaluate your own church the same way.

Can you observe any people with disabilities serving in ministry?

> In leadership?

Are there wheelchair users in the isle or all lined along the back? Are people with disabilities being segregated? Notate your observations.

_____

_____

_____

_____

_____

_____

_____

_____

_____

_____

_____

Now look at your church's communication or promotional materials. Does their mission statement or other materials sound like they welcome everyone, including people with disabilities? Is this inclusiveness apparent? Why? Why not?

_____

_____

_____

_____

_____

Did you speak with anyone about disabilities ministry? What was the response?

_____

_____

_____

_____

_____

_____

_____

2: Inclusive Culture

My brothers and sisters, believers in our glorious Lord Jesus Christ must not show favoritism. Suppose a man comes into your meeting wearing gold ring and fine clothes, and a poor man in filthy old clothes also comes in. If you show special attention to the man wearing fine clothes and say, "Here's a good seat for you," but say to the poor man, "You stand there" or "Sit on the floor by my feet," have you not discriminated among yourselves and become judges with evil thoughts?

James 2:1-4

Read the scripture closely. Does your church practice segregation?? Who is welcome at your church? What makes you so sure? What evidence do you have to prove this?

_____

_____

_____

_____

Axis Dance Company website & video

http://www.axisdance.org

https://www.youtube.com/watch?v=OUHgMtyjT-4

Describe the inclusive culture of Axis Dance Company. How can the church or your organization emulate this culture?

_____

_____

_____

_____

_____

Visit an agency that works with people with physical, mental, emotional, or educational disabilities. Collect and read information about the agency's activities. Learn about opportunities its members/clients have for training, employment, and education. Document your observations.

_____

_____

_____

DEBBIE MALONE

3: Barriers

Therefore, let us stop passing judgment on one another. Instead, make up your mind not to put any stumbling block or obstacle in the way of a brother or sister.

Romans 14:13

Identify your personal prejudices.

What are your real attitudes and fears about people with disabilities?

_____

_____

_____

_____

_____

_____

Answer these questions honestly (adapted from the ABA Commission on Disability Rights. Implicit Biases & People with Disabilities.)

1. When you think of a person with a disability, do you focus on the things the person can do or cannot do? Where do you get the information on which you base your views? Did you ask or observe the person with a disability?

_____

_____

_____

_____

_____

_____

_____

2. Do you think of a person with a disability as working in certain careers? If so, which careers and why?

_____

_____

_____

_____

_____

3. When you think of a person with a disability, do you have sympathy or feel pity for the person?

_____

_____

_____

_____

4. When you meet a person with a disability, do you see the person's disability before you see the person?

_____

_____

_____

_____

5. Do you think about people with disabilities as a group or as individuals? If as a group, what characteristics do you think people with disabilities share?

_____

_____

_____

_____

6. Do you consider people with disabilities as different from people without disabilities? If so, how are they different?

_____

_____

_____

_____

7. Do you believe that the lives of people with disabilities are different from the lives of people without disabilities? If so, how are they different?

_____

_____

_____

_____

8. Do you use terms (e.g., "normal" or "able-bodied") to differentiate between people without disabilities and people with disabilities?

_____

_____

_____

_____

9. Do you speak to and interact with people with disabilities differently than you do with people without disabilities? If so, how and why?

_____

_____

_____

_____

10. Do you perceive people with disabilities as dependent compared to people without disabilities? Do you base your belief on personal experiences or other sources? If the latter, what are the sources?

_____

_____

_____

_____

11. Would you describe persons with disabilities as brave, courageous, inspirational, superhuman, and heroic? If so, why?

_____

_____

_____

12. Do you perceive people with disabilities as productive or competent as people without disabilities? If so, why?

_____

_____

_____

_____

13. Do you view people with disabilities as too costly for employers to hire? If so, please explain.

_____

_____

_____

_____

14. Do you view disability as an abnormality or sickness or as a challenge that needs to be overcome or corrected? When you see a person with a disability, do you automatically want to help them?

_____

_____

_____

_____

15. Do you think workers with disabilities receive special advantages or are held to a lesser standard than workers without disabilities?

_____

_____

_____

_____

Specific Disabilities

1. Do you perceive persons with mental illness as violent or dangerous? If so, based on what information?

_____

_____

_____

2.   Do you view people with intellectual disabilities or developmental disabilities as being dependent on others to care for them? As being kind and generous? As being innocent and sweet-natured?

_____

_____

_____

3.   Do you think all blind people have a keener sense of smell and hearing? Why?

_____

_____

_____

4. Do you think people with cerebral palsy have cognitive impairments as well?

_____

_____

_____

5. Do you view people with hidden impairments such as learning disabilities, arthritis, and heart conditions as having a disability?

_____

_____

_____

6. Do you think all blind people read braille? Why?

_____

_____

_____

DEBBIE MALONE

4: People First Language

The words of the reckless pierce like swords, but the tongue of the wise brings healing.

Proverbs 12:18

For one week write down what you think or say that may be hurtful toward people with disabilities. What is encouraging?

_____

_____

_____

_____

_____

_____

Write alternative positive statements. Keep the list with you as a reminder.

_____

_____

_____

_____

_____

_____

_____

_____

_____

_____

_____

_____

_____

_____

Print or write the people first chart below. Change your speaking patterns to reflect people first language every day.

People First Language	Language to Avoid
Person with a disability	The disabled, handicapped
Person without a disability	Normal person, healthy person
Person with an intellectual, cognitive, developmental disability	Retarded, slow, simple, moronic, defective or retarded, afflicted, special person
Person with an emotional or behavioral disability, person with a mental health or a psychiatric disability	Insane, crazy, psycho, maniac, nuts
Person who is hard of hearing	Hearing impaired, suffers a hearing loss
Person who is deaf	Deaf and dumb, mute
Person who is blind/visually impaired	The blind
Person who has a communication disorder, is unable to speak, or uses a device to speak	Mute, dumb
Person who uses a wheelchair	Confined or restricted to a wheelchair, wheelchair bound
Person with a physical disability	Crippled, lame, deformed, invalid, spastic
Person with epilepsy or seizure disorder	Epileptic
Person with multiple sclerosis	Afflicted by MS
Person with cerebral palsy	CP victim
Accessible parking or bathrooms	Handicapped parking or bathroom
Person of short stature	Midget
Person with Down syndrome	Mongoloid
Person who is successful, productive	Has overcome his/her disability, is courageous

Read newspaper articles or listen to news about someone or a group of people with disabilities. Observe language. Take notes.

_____

_____

_____

_____

_____

_____

_____

_____

_____

_____

_____

_____

_____

5: Etiquette

Be devoted to one another in love. Honor one another above yourselves.

Romans 12:10

Read etiquette handout (Unlikely Dancer 2, p53-56 or https://www.umdisabilityministries.org/welcoming/etiquette.html.). Pick one item from each category or one category to change each week. Note your successes and struggles.

_____

_____

_____

_____

_____

_____

Observe how people are treated in stores, restaurants, etc. As you interact with people with disabilities, practice etiquette at work, in the community, and at church. If people with disabilities attend church, practice proper disability etiquette

_____

_____

_____

_____

_____

_____

_____

_____

_____

_____

_____

6: Training

And this is my prayer: that your love may abound more and more in knowledge and depth of insight,

Philippians 1:9

How does this scripture relate to disability inclusion?

_____

_____

_____

_____

_____

_____

Learn about welcoming people with disabilities in the church.

Disability Sensitivity Training Video

https://www.youtube.com/watch?v=Gv1aDEFlXq8

Disability Awareness, Sensitivity and Practical Inclusion Training

https://www.youtube.com/watch?v=b_GO4beTspA

DISABILITY AWARENESS FILM | Basingstoke & District Disability Forum

https://www.youtube.com/watch?v=aJssu_PAw4w

Watch the videos and take notes

_____

_____

_____

_____

_____

_____

_____

_____

_____

DEBBIE MALONE

Part II: Keep Us

Belonging

And let us consider one another to provoke unto love and to good works: Not forsaking the assembling of ourselves together, as the manner of some is; but exhorting one another: and so much the more, as ye see the day approaching.

Hebrews 10:24-25

Disability Ministry in the Church | Mini Documentary

https://www.youtube.com/watch?v=cOguNeLUWfA&t=359s

Watch video and write notes for yourself.

_____

_____

_____

_____

_____

_____

_____

_____

_____

_____

_____

_____

_____

_____

_____

_____

7: Heart

The goal of this command is love, which comes from a pure heart and a good conscience and a sincere faith.

1 Timothy 1:5

Examine your heart. Reveal your inner attitude toward people with disabilities.

_____

_____

_____

_____

_____

_____

While at church, do you sit with or carry on conversations with people who are different? Why? Why not?

_____

_____

_____

_____

_____

Are you embarrassed to let others see you engaging and befriending those people who not only may look different, but may act different?

_____

_____

_____

_____

Do you encourage others to be themselves or do you try to get them to fit into a mold of acceptable church behavior?

_____

_____

_____

_____

Do you engage conversations with people with disabilities only at church? Do you avoid people with disabilities in the community?

_____

_____

_____

_____

_____

Where do you fall in the stages? What has influenced your attitude. Be honest.

5 Stages: The Journey of Disability Attitudes

STAGE 1: IGNORANCE

STAGE 2: PITY

STAGE 3: CARE

STAGE 4: FRIENDSHIP

STAGE 5: CO-LABORERS

_____

_____

_____

_____

_____

Write an action plan for yourself. How will you go to the next level? Be specific. Write personal goals.

_____

_____

_____

_____

_____

_____

_____

_____

_____

_____

_____

_____

_____

Access the following resources. Try to discover attitudinal barriers around you no matter how subtle they appear. Make notes

Handout: Attitudinal Barriers. Retrieved from UUA.org: https://www.uua.org/sites/live-new.uua.org/files/handout_attitudinal_barriers.pdf

Attitudinal Barriers for People with Disabilities. Retrieved from NCWD: http://www.ncwd-youth.info/publications/attitudinal-barriers-for-people-with-disabilities/

_____

_____

_____

_____

_____

_____

_____

_____

_____

_____

What is your church's opinion about people with disabilities? Where does your church fall in the phases of disability inclusion? Do the actions coincide with the church's promotional matereials?

_____

_____

_____

_____

_____

_____

_____

_____

_____

_____

_____

_____

_____

Perform the assessment, then devise a plan to bring awareness and eliminate negative attitudes.

Attitude Barrier Assessment:	Y	N	Comments
People with disabilities and their caregivers have been asked whether they feel welcome in worship, leadership, and church programs.			
Our church is intentional about engaging people with disabilities in all aspects of church life. People with disabilities serve on church committees or in other leadership roles.			
Our church has a church disability advocate and/or committee.			
Ushers, teachers, and youth leaders/mentors have been instructed regarding appropriate ways to greet and respond to the needs of people with disabilities.			
Our church has adopted a Church Policy on Disabilities.			
Church leaders work with people with disabilities and caregivers so that needs are addressed, including pastoral care.			
Are persons with disabilities being included in this audit process?			
Is the congregation made aware that one in five persons lives with a disability and one in four persons experiences a mental health concern over a lifetime?			
Does the church offer regular educational opportunities for congregants through			

newsletters, information sessions, sermons, and small group discussions aimed at awareness of the breadth of disabilities?		
Are members willing to thoughtfully include persons with disabilities in leadership boards and committees, study, worship services, and recreational activities?		
Do members acknowledge that inclusion is more than ramps, restrooms, and parking places?		
Is sensitivity training required for ushers, greeters, church staff, and others who encounter persons with disabilities?		

$8.$ Friendships

A new command I give you: Love one another. As I have loved you, so you must love one another. By this everyone will know that you are my disciples, if you love one another."

John 13:34-35

Think about the people you know. Are you making any effort to befriend anyone with disabilities? Who? What efforts have you made?

_____

_____

_____

_____

_____

_____

_____

Do any of your friends have disabilities? Are they visible or hidden? Are you uncomfortable with them in public? Do you go to each other's homes for dinner or to just hang out and have fun?

_____

_____

_____

_____

_____

Pick one family or person with a disability. Try to find a family or person that you would naturally befriend. Do you have similar interests? Do you have children who are similar ages? Invite them to spend time with you. Go for coffee. Go shopping. Get to know each other. Make not of the experiences, including your feelings about the family.

_____

_____

_____

_____

_____

_____

Write about the person you are choosing to befriend. Describe your initial experiences together. How is it developing? How does the disability affect the relationship? How does the disability affect what activities you can participate in? Do you see God in the friendship? Are both of you encouraged with the time you spend together?

_____

_____

_____

_____

_____

_____

_____

_____

_____

9: ADA

Let everyone be subject to the governing authorities, for there is no authority except that which God has established. The authorities that exist have been established by God. Consequently, whoever rebels against the authority is rebelling against what God has instituted, and those who do so will bring judgment on themselves.

Romans 13:1-2

Does an outside group or organization operate a program within your building? If the answer is yes, then the church may be obligated under Title III of the ADA. Title III information can be found at https://www.ada.gov/ada_title_III.htm.

_____

_____

_____

_____

Does your church employ more than 15 people? If the answer is yes, then the church would be obligated under Title I of the ADA. Information can be found at https://www.ada.gov/ada_title_I.htm.

_____

_____

_____

_____

_____

_____

Are there situations in your church that must comply with the Americans with Disabilities Act (ADA) regulations?

_____

_____

_____

_____

_____

Many places of worship voluntarily comply with ADA regulations to provide a more inclusive environment. When making any building upgrades, it is a good time to include accessibility features. Also, local building codes may require accessibility. Check with the church's lawyer and building inspectors for more information.

Is your church considering upgrading any part of the building now or in the future? Give input about the need for accessibility. Write about your efforts and the response. Should more be done? How will you advocate for people with disabilities?

_____

_____

_____

_____

_____

_____

_____

_____

_____

_____

_____

10: Physical Accessibility

And it will be said: "Build up, build up, prepare the road!
Remove the obstacles out of the way of my people."

Isaiah 57:14

Take a walk around your church building and grounds. Use the following checklist to discover any physical obstacles. In the comments section write your opinion about the item. Is it really needed? What is the feasibility of the problem being corrected?

Church Accessibility Checklist

Parking Lot & Building Entrance:	Y	N	Comments:
Are 1 in 25 parking spaces handicap accessible?			
Are at least 1 of the handicap parking spaces van accessible?			
Is it possible to get from a parked car into the building without using stairs?			
Do curbs on the route have curb cuts at drives, parking, and drop offs?			
Is the main entrance accessible?			
Do all inaccessible entrances have signs indicating the location of the nearest accessible entrance?			
Do any platforms extend at least 1' beyond each side of the doorway?			
Are parking spaces at least 132" with a 60"aisle (universal guidelines)?			
Are walkways and curb cuts clearly marked?			
Do walkways and curb cuts have non-slip surfaces?			
Are ramps a minimum of 36" in width, extending one foot in length for every inch of rise (1':12" ratio) and have handrails on at least one side if over 6' in length?			
Is there a level rest platform at least 5' long for every 30" of ramp rise and a 5' x 5' platform at changes of direction?			
Entrances and hallways are free from barriers that can impede a wheelchair (door bases, grates, thick mats).			
Doors:			
Do all doors open completely?			
Are door thresholds no more than ½ inch in height?			
Do doors have lever type hardware, panic bars or automatic door openers?			
Can doors be opened with exerting 5 pounds of pressure or less?			

Stairs:			
Are the edges of stairs and raised cracks in sidewalks' edges painted with a contrasting color (often yellow) so people with low vision can see and be safe?			
Do they have non-slip surfaces?			
Is there good lighting for stairways?			
Are stairways at least 44 inches wide with handrails on both sides?			
Can handrails support at least 250 pounds?			
Do handrails on stairs extend one foot at the bottom and top of stairs?			
Elevators and Lifts:			
If the facility has multiple stories, are there elevators?			
Are the elevators easy to locate?			
Is there an elevator or chair lift for access to the sanctuary and all major areas?			
Are controls placed 54 inches or less from the floor, reachable from a wheelchair?			
Are Braille plaques on elevator control panels?			
Restrooms:			
Is an accessible restroom located on every floor?			
Do you have an adult sized changing table in a restroom/private space?			
Is there at least one stall that is 36" wide or the preferred 42"?			
Do stalls have a turning space of 5'X5' for easy wheelchair use?			
Are grab bars securely fastened to the wall on each side?			
Is the countertop or sink top no more than 34" above the floor?			
Is there at least 27" from the floor to the bottom of the countertop or sink?			
Are soap dispensers no higher than 44" from the floor?			
Are there lever type faucet controls and hardware on the doors?			
Water Fountain:			

Does each floor have a disability accessible water fountain?		
Is the top rim of the water fountain between 30"-34" above the floor or a drinking cup dispenser no higher than 40"?		
Signage:		
Are signage letters and numbers sized for optimal reading at the required distances?		
Are permanent signs located on the walls adjacent to the door's latch side or on the nearest wall?		
Can a person approach the signs within 3" without running into an object standing in a swinging doorway		
Is there braille to identify rooms, elevators, etc.?		
Is there a slightly raised & brightly colored abrasive strip to warn of open staircases?		
Are there are fire alarm systems with both flashing lights and audible signals?		
Worship Center:		
Are sound levels adequate for persons with hearing impairments?		
Can the sound be amplified with an induction loop or mini-broadcasting system?		
Is lighting adequate to enable persons to worship?		
Can speakers or interpreters be easily seen without shadows?		
Are large print Bibles, hymnals and bulletins available?		
Are an adequate number of wheelchair spaces provided? *Suggested 1 per 25 seats.*		
Are wheelchair spaces dispersed to allow location choices and viewing angles equivalent to other seating?		
Can people take communion without climbing stairs?		
Do ramps have smooth-surfaced handrails on both sides?		

Is at least at least one primary entrance usable by individuals in wheelchairs?		
Are doorway openings 36" wide or more?		
Are doors operable by a single effort?		
Are there automatic doors?		
Are doors sills safe and free from safe inclines or abrupt changes?		
Is seating space with extra leg room available for those with crutches, braces, walkers, etc.?		
Are ushers familiar with special needs and willing to assist as needed?		
Classrooms:		
Are door thresholds no higher than one half inch?		
Is there excellent lighting in all areas?		
Are the following available for children: soft blocks for children having behavioral issues; tactile signage on furniture, learning centers, doors, etc.; wheelchair lap table for a child in a wheelchair who cannot pull up to a child size table?		
Are doorway openings 36" wide or more?		
Is there an accessible desk/table space in each classroom (with no attached chair)?		
Is there an easily accessible wheelchair route to the front of the classroom?		
Additional Items:		
Does the church own a wheelchair accessible van?		
Does the church provide transportation for people who are unable to drive?		
Coats racks can be accessed by all people.		
Church mailboxes are accessible		

For more detailed specifications download the ADA Accessibility Checklist from https://www.adachecklist.org/doc/fullchecklist/ada-checklist.pdf.

DEBBIE MALONE

11: Equipment and Devices

And he hath filled him with the spirit of God, in wisdom, in understanding, and in knowledge, and in all manner of workmanship; And to devise curious works, to work in gold, and in silver, and in brass,

Exodus 35:31-32

Ask people with disabilities (or a family member if the person cannot speak for him/herself) if there is any equipment or devices that the church could provide that would be helpful. Wheelchairs and assistive listening devices are common. Perhaps a table that is the right height to accommodate a wheelchair may be requested. Be willing to listen no matter what is requested. List them and look for ways to provide them.

Let the family know that you are doing research and can't promise anything, but you will try. It is better to be honest than to make promises you cannot keep.

_____

_____

Make an appointment with the director or a knowledgeable case manager at your local Independent Living Center. (http://www.ilru.org/projects/cil-net/cil-center-and-association-directory) Ask about the center. What services do they offer? Get copies of their materials to review later.

Ask about the types of equipment that would be advisable to have on-hand. Perhaps mentioning that you are thinking about having wheelchair or two and some assistive listening devices. Are there places that have donations? Would a church qualify to receive any equipment? Follow up on the recommendations. Keep the connections. The ILC will be a good resource in the future.

_____

_____

_____

_____

_____

_____

_____

_____

_____

12: Creativity

And he hath filled him with the spirit of God, in wisdom, in understanding, and in knowledge, and in all manner of workmanship; And to devise curious works, to work in gold, and in silver, and in brass, And in the cutting of stones, to set them, and in carving of wood, to make any manner of cunning work.

Exodus 35:31-33

Look around your environment. List five items that are the result of a creative inventor. Research the inventor and the circumstances that caused the need for creativity.

_____

_____

_____

_____

Speak with three different people with disabilities. Learn about each person's experiences and the activities in which this person likes to participate. Summarize the discussion.

_____

_____

_____

_____

_____

_____

_____

_____

_____

_____

_____

_____

_____

Discuss typical accommodations that he/she has needed.

_____

_____

_____

_____

_____

_____

Ask about any situation that required a creative solution. Consider different ways of accomplishing a task, creative uses of common items, and the creation of new devices.

_____

_____

_____

_____

_____

_____

_____

13: Technology and Communication

"Thou shalt not curse the deaf, nor put a stumbling block before the blind, but shalt fear thy God: I am the LORD."

Leviticus 19:14

Write a list of possible stumbling blocks in the technology and the communication ministries of your church or organization.

_____

_____

_____

_____

_____

Perform a Technology and Communication Accessibility assessment.

Technology and Communication Accessibility Assessment			
Communication:	**Y**	**N**	**Comments**
Our church has assistive listening devices (infrared, hearing loop, FM) available for people with hearing impairments.			
Sign-language interpretation is provided when prior arrangements have been made.			
Overall lighting is adequate for signing and speech reading, or for individuals with low vision.			
Songbooks, Bibles, bulletins, newsletters, and handouts are available in alternative formats such as large print, audio, and digital (also Braille, when requested in advance).			
Information about alternate format materials is prominently displayed. readily accessible.			
Alternate format materials are readily available.			
Copies of the day's sermon and spoken elements of worship are available for people with impaired hearing?			
Are cassettes or CDs of services and other events available?			
Are printed sermons available?			
Are large print bulletins, hymnals (or printed lyrics), and Bibles available?			
Are large print handouts and printed PowerPoint slides available?			
Are volunteers available to read bulletins, lyrics, and Bibles when needed if a Braille embosser is not available?			
Technology:			
Is the website accessible for users of assistive technology?			
Is captioning used with all visual projection.			
Do all photographs and illustrations (including text printed as			

images) on websites and social media have an "alt-text."			
Is audio description used for all videos?			
Is there appropriate color contrast between text and background?			
Is the background behind text solid?			
Does each link on a webpage describe what that link is to (not using "click here")?			
Has the website passed accessibility testing?			
Are all emails, newsletters, outreach materials available in alternate formats?			
Is there signage and notice of availability of all assistive equipment and alternate format materials?			

DEBBIE MALONE

14: Teaching Methods

I will instruct you and teach you in the way you should go; I will counsel you with my loving eye on you.

Psalm 32:8

Review *A Sampling of Special Needs Curriculum and Resources.*
https://irresistiblechurch.org/wp-content/uploads/2014/02/ASamplingofSpecialNeedsCurriculumandResources-final.pdf

_____

_____

_____

_____

_____

Review the *UDL Guidelines*. http://udlguidelines.cast.org/

_____

_____

_____

_____

_____

Observe each church class (Sunday school classes, Bible study). Evaluate the teaching methods using the Universal Design for Learning Guidelines and the ideas from *A Sampling of Special Needs Curriculum and Resources.* Describe your observations, positive and negative.

_____

_____

_____

_____

_____

_____

_____

Speak with students and/or parents. What is working? What does not work? Are the students learning? Are there any recommendations?

_____

_____

_____

_____

_____

_____

_____

_____

_____

_____

_____

The teachers should get to know their students and devise strategies to teach to their strengths. Ask the teachers to have all the parents fill out an intake form. Create your own form or use the following example from JoniandFriends.org, the Irresistible Church Series.

[Insert Church Name] Special Needs Parent Intake Form

These questions allow us to provide the best experience and safest environment for all our friends within the ministry. Our church leaders and ministry volunteers will respect your family's right to privacy. Any information shared is communicated directly with those caring for your family member and only on a "need to know" basis. If you have any questions, please contact [Insert Name] for more information.

Child's Name: _____

DOB: _____

Mother's Name _____

Phone #_____

Live at home? Y N

Address _____City _____

        ZIP _____

Email _____

Alternate Phone # _____

Father's Name _____

Phone # _____

Live at home? Y   N

Address _____City _____

     ZIP _____

Email _____

Alternate Phone # _____

Siblings?

Name _____ Age _____

Name _____ Age _____

Name _____ Age _____

Name _____ Age _____

Allergies/Food Sensitivities: ☐Yes ☐ No

If yes, please explain _____

_____

Are the allergies life threatening?   ☐ Yes ☐ No

   EPI Pen? ☐ Yes ☐ No

Food/drinks to avoid: _____

_____

Is assistance needed for eating/drinking? ☐ Yes ☐ No

Prone to Seizures: ☐ Yes ☐ No Other Medical Concerns: ____

_____

_____

_____

Toileting Needs: ☐ Independent   ☐ Needs Assistance
   ☐ Wears Diapers

Signs, Gestures, Words to Indicate Toileting Needs _____

_____

_____

Medication: ☐ Yes ☐ No Type and Purpose: _____

_____

_____

Main Mode(s) of Communication: ☐ Verbal ☐ Visual Supports
   ☐ Sign Language   ☐ Digital Devices

My child is independent with _____

_____

_____

My child needs assistance with _____

_____

_____

My child is uncomfortable with or has sensitivities to _____

_____

_____

Behavior concerns to be aware of: _____

_____

_____

Trigger-points for frustration/resistance: _____

_____

_____

Calming tools and aids: _____

_____

_____

Behaviors that may communicate a specific need (please indicate the
need where appropriate): _____

_____

_____

Classroom situations you wish to be contacted about: _____

_____

_____

_____

My child loves to _____

_____

_____

Enjoys music? ☐ Yes ☐ No

Enjoys arts & crafts? ☐ Yes ☐ No

Outside play? ☐ Yes ☐ No

Writing? ☐ Yes ☐ No   Reading? ☐Yes ☐ No

Please describe your child's understanding of and relationship with God: _____

_____

_____

Goals for your child at church: _____

_____

_____

Ideas for church to better serve your family: _____

_____

_____

Additional thoughts or comments: _____

_____

_____

_____

_____

15: Transportation

"The servant came back and reported this to his master. Then the owner of the house became angry and ordered his servant, 'Go out quickly into the streets and alleys of the town and bring in the poor, the crippled, the blind and the lame.'

"'Sir,' the servant said, 'what you ordered has been done, but there is still room.'

"Then the master told his servant, 'Go out to the roads and country lanes and compel them to come in, so that my house will be full.

Luke 14: 15-24

Research transportation alternatives in your area. You may want to consider the local public transit authority, taxicabs, and individual volunteers. Senior centers, rehabilitation agencies, Independent living centers, and your city or county ADA coordinator are valuable resources. Consider the types of vehicles and what types of disabilities are accommodated. Consider cost, scheduling, convenience, and reliability. Keep a record of your results.

_____

_____

_____

_____

_____

_____

_____

Now research wheelchair accessible vehicles. Determine features and costs.

_____

_____

_____

_____

_____

_____

Bring all research results to your disability ministry leader (if you have one) or pastor. Discuss the best alternatives for your church. Plan to provide increasingly reliable, inexpensive transportation that would allow more people with disabilities to attend services and activities. Start a transportation ministry or add to one that already exists.

Bonus Challenge: If you drive do not drive anywhere for one month. You cannot get rides from anyone in your household. Rely on public transportation, taxis, Uber, friends, or co-workers. Keep a journal. It can be written, videoed, recorded. Describe the process of getting rides. Share your feelings. Determine the other person's attitudes.

_____

_____

_____

_____

_____

_____

_____

_____

_____

_____

_____

Anticipate what would happen if your situation was permanent. Every three to four months you will need replace the rides from friends, co-workers, and family (not of your household). Describe the anticipation, fear, and uncertainty of this prospect.

_____

_____

_____

_____

_____

_____

_____

_____

_____

_____

_____

_____

DEBBIE MALONE

16: Service Dogs

For every kind of beast and bird, of reptile and sea creature, can be tamed and has been tamed by mankind.

James 3:7

Research a local service dog or guide dog training facility. Make an appointment to visit. Come prepared with questions. What did you learn? What are your observations?

_____

_____

_____

_____

_____

_____

Interview someone with a service dog or guide dog. Get to know the lifestyle associated with having a service animal. What are the benefits? What are the challenges?

_____

_____

_____

_____

_____

_____

Interview leaders of your church concerning service dogs. What is their opinion? Would they prefer to not have service dogs in the sanctuary, fellowship hall, classrooms, or café? How do they feel about service dogs riding in church vehicles? Individual private vehicles?

_____

_____

_____

_____

_____

_____

Develop a service dog module for a disability awareness workshop. Make it interesting and informative. Include an etiquette section about service dogs and guide dogs.

_____

_____

_____

_____

_____

_____

_____

_____

_____

_____

17: Recreation

And also that every man should eat and drink, and enjoy
the good of all his labour, it is the gift of God.

Ecclesiastes 3:13

What types of activities do you (and your family) enjoy? Think about
indoor and outdoor games, sports, events. Write a list.

_____

_____

_____

_____

_____

_____

_____

What would prevent you from inviting a family that has a member with a disability to join your family on an outing? Examine your own concerns. Are you afraid there may be an accident? Perhaps the individual with the disability may be too slow. Are you impatient about the extra care that may be required? Be honest with yourself.

_____

_____

_____

_____

_____

_____

_____

_____

_____

_____

_____

Now, despite your reservations extend an invitation. Find out what the other family might like to do for fun. Plan a joint recreational activity together.

_____

_____

_____

_____

Research local adaptive sports activities. Many parks and recreation departments have developed specialized programs. Can you incorporate them into church recreational activities? Your family's activities?

_____

_____

_____

_____

_____

_____

_____

_____

_____

Are people and families affected by disability attending church activities outside of the building? Why? Why not? If you do not know, ask. Record you answers. Formulate a plan for inclusive recreational activities.

_____

_____

_____

_____

_____

_____

_____

_____

_____

18: Additional Considerations

Write a policy concerning fragrances. Should the church should use only unscented products, such as cleaning products and candles? Should the entire building be a fragrance-free facility or only certain areas or rooms?

_____

_____

_____

_____

_____

_____

_____

Conduct this additional assessment.

Leadership:	Y	N	Comments
Do the pastor and the church staff receive training in disability awareness?			
Are the pastor and pastoral visitors aware they should request an interpreter or communication materials when visiting persons with communication-based disabilities?			
Do teachers receive sensitivity training for working with persons with disabilities, including adapting materials?			
Are reimbursements available for additional expenses such as accessible transportation, rental of mobility, audio, interpreting or other equipment as needed for disabled persons who represent the church at meetings, retreats, conferences?			
Are reasonable accommodations made when persons with disabilities are in any worship leadership capacity, i.e. choir members, readers, musicians?			
Miscellaneous:			
Signs, websites, or bulletin boards offer evidence that people with visible and hidden disabilities are welcome and included in the life of the congregation, e.g. through brochures, photos,			
Disruptions are accepted and incorporated into worship			
Needs of people on special diets are considered when food is offered, including gluten-free & alcohol-free communion elements			
"Buddy" system offered for individuals needing 1:1 assistance			

Part III: Use Us

Serving

For we are God's handiwork, created in Christ Jesus to do good works, which God prepared in advance for us to do.

Ephesians 2:10

Observe inclusiveness within your organization. Are people with disabilities leaders? Does the advertising show people with disabilities in various roles amid the organization/church? How can you help facilitate change?

_____

_____

_____

_____

Are church events and activities accessible for all who want to participate? Describe your observations, positive and negative.

_____

_____

_____

_____

_____

_____

_____

_____

_____

_____

_____

_____

_____

19: Evangelism, Discipleship, and Participation

Then Jesus said to his host, "When you give a luncheon or dinner, do not invite your friends, your brothers or sisters, your relatives, or your rich neighbors; if you do, they may invite you back and so you will be repaid. But when you give a banquet, invite the poor, the crippled, the lame, the blind, and you will be blessed. Although they cannot repay you, you will be repaid at the resurrection of the righteous."

Luke 14:12-14

Develop a plan to intentionally evangelize people with disabilities.

1. Research (record your findings)
    a. demographics of your community
    b. local agencies that serve people with disabilities
2. Prepare the congregation to receive people with disabilities (discuss best approaches with leadership)
    a. Disability Awareness Sunday
    b. Sermon Series
    c. Workshop

3. Engage in the community
   a. Plan to go where the people are. Be creative.
   b. Host events to bring in people with disabilities. Be creative.

Develop discipleship opportunities.

    1. Recruit individuals who will be willing and able to mentor people with disabilities.

    2. Provide training to mentors, including special considerations of discipling people with disabilities.

    3. Provide training and growth opportunities for people with disabilities.

    4. Identify opportunities for everyone affected by disability to serve. Make a list. Place person's name next to each opportunity as appropriate.

_____

_____

_____

_____

_____

_____

_____

_____

_____

_____

_____

_____

_____

_____

_____

_____

_____

_____

_____

_____

_____

_____

_____

_____

Develop service opportunities.

    1. Identify gifts and talents of each person affected by disability.

    2. Place individuals in positions of service, including leadership roles.

_____

_____

_____

_____

_____

_____

_____

_____

_____

_____

_____

_____

_____

_____

_____

_____

_____

_____

_____

_____

_____

_____

_____

_____

_____

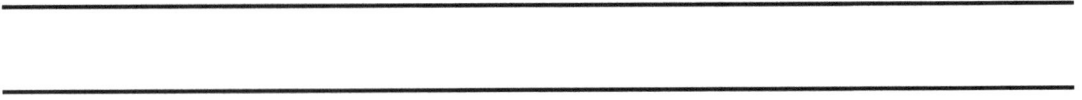

20: Establishing a Disability Ministry

We ought therefore to show hospitality to such people so that we may work together for the truth.

3 John 8

Organize a team. Develop a meeting schedule.

_____

_____

_____

_____

_____

_____

_____

Train the team. Include barriers, disability etiquette, and language first. Schedule the training.

_____

_____

_____

_____

_____

_____

_____

_____

_____

_____

_____

_____

Gather information.

1. Survey/questionnaire for individuals in congregation
2. Conversations with families affected by disability.
3. Previously completed research about the population of the community and agencies serving people with disabilities.

Now, summarize the results and prioritize the needs.

_____

_____

_____

_____

_____

_____

_____

_____

_____

_____

_____

Meet the needs of the people you already have. Make note of those requests and how they were met. Note the dates of the request and the fulfillment date. Determine the amount of time that elapsed between the two dates. Was this reasonable or is there more work to be done in this area. Keep track of all the requests.

Action Plan for Meeting Immediate Needs		
Need/date	Action plan	Completed/date

Sample congregation survey.

CHURCH SURVEY

Part of the growth to becoming *Irresistible* is the ability to honestly reflect upon where we are and where we need to go. Please take a few moments to fill out this survey – it will help church leadership to determine the best "next steps" in creating a special needs ministry.

5 Stages* – Please mark both where you are & where your church is related to how you see, believe about and respond to individuals affected by disability.

Me	Church	
		Ignorance – God doesn't care, individual is sinful or broken, God is not involved
		Pity – I am blessed, grateful that I am not affected, they need me to provide value
		Care – created in God's image, they have value, I support showing love
		Friendship – spend time with individuals, I am blessed by my friend, my life is better
		Co-Laborers – called to serve & love God, we all give & receive, encourage together

Are any members of your family affected by disability?   Yes   No
If yes, please briefly describe.

Do your family members attend church regularly?   Yes   No
How could our church better serve in this area?

If one or more of your family members are children, do they regularly attend class?
        Yes   No

How could we better serve and make the classrooms more accessible?

What could be done to better serve and support your family?

If your family would like to attend our church, what practical changes should be made?

  More accessible parking   Large-print Bibles
  Better lighting   Better sound equipment
  Sign-language interpreter   Appropriate wheelchair space
  Class for adults with developmental disabilities
  Special childcare for Services

  Other

Outside of regular weekend services, please mark which ministries would benefit your family.

☐ Regular Date Nights

☐ Family Support groups

☐ Dad/s Day Out

☐ Mom's Morning Out

☐ Child/youth-based events

☐ Financial Planning, support services

The Growth of a Ministry- We are in the beginning stages of growing a special needs ministry with the goal of becoming an *Irresistible Church* in our community. To accomplish this goal, we need you. Would you please consider the following areas of ministry need and mark any places you feel God is calling you to serve in and make a difference through this ministry?

☐ I would like to be part of the leadership and planning a team.

☐ I would like to become a sidekick for our children and youth ministries.

☐ I would like to serve on Date Nights on a monthly basis.

☐ I am trained in special needs through medical, psychological, or other fields and am interested in assisting, training, intake, etc.

☐ I am interested in serving as needed.

Name_____

Phone_____

Address_____

City_____ State_____ Zip_____

Family Member (including ae of child)

_____

Additional Comments:

DEBBIE MALONE

$\mathcal{21:}$ Transition Plan

Then the LORD replied: "Write down the revelation and make it plain on tablets so that a herald may run with it.

Habakkuk 2:2

Start Small. We met the current needs in the last chapter.

Using your priority list from the last section, make a specific plan to achieve full inclusion. Each church/agency plan will have different priorities and resources.

_____

_____

_____

_____

Short term goals (three months or under). List goals and formulate a plan, including a completion date goal.

Short-Term Goals			
Item	Action plan	Goal date	Complete date

Long Range goals. List and formulate a plan, including fundraising ideas if needed.

Long-Term Goals			
Item	Action plan	Goal date	Complete date

Here is another idea. You may want to combine the long- and short-term goals in one form. Action plans usually require more space than provided. Do what works for you and your church leadership.

Transition Plan: Toward Full Inclusion				
Item	Responsible person	Goal date	Completion date	Action Plan

DEBBIE MALONE

22: Provision

But my God shall supply all your need according to his riches in glory by Christ Jesus.

Philippians 4:19

Describe an unusual situation, in which God provided for you and your family. Keep it in a place where you can be reminded of Jehovah Jirah.

As a team discuss possible ways to raise money. Be creative. Use social media, websites, and any means of communicating with members and with the community

Seek approval from the pastor and leaders. Some ideas may not fit well with your church's beliefs.

Some considerations may be:
1. Crowdfunding
2. Peer-to-Peer Fundraising
3. Create a Text-to-Give Campaign
4. T-shirt Fundraising
5. Shoe Drive
6. Matching Gifts

7. Giving Kiosks
8. Volunteer Grants
9. Host a Sing-along
10. Use Church Newsletter
11. Cookbooks
12. Create and Sell Calendars
13. Walk-a-Thons
14. Host a Movie Night
15. Talent Show

These are just a few ideas from church fundraising websites. Find ones that will compliment your church culture and belief system.

Before seeking grants, the church should become a 501c3 organization with the IRS. This establishes your church as a charitable organization which allows you to apply for many types of funding.

Research local, state and private sources.

Here are some places to start.

1. Grants.gov
2. Urban Ministry Grants
3. Grants for Nonprofits: Religion and Social Change
4. Churchgrants.org
5. Local Foundations
6. Walmart Foundation
7. FundsnetServices.com

Develop a fundraising plan. Pray and seek God's direction. Use the following space to jot down notes and get organized.

_____

_____

_____

_____

_____

_____

_____

_____

_____

_____

_____

_____

_____

Fundraising can be a daunting task. Be creative. Use available resources. Perhaps a local high school or trade school provides on-site experience for its students. With teacher supervision, construction, plumbing, electricity, and other trades could be utilized inexpensively.

Think out of the box. Pray and welcome god's direction. He will provide in unexpected ways

.

23: Personal Calling

Therefore, my brothers and sisters, make every effort to confirm your calling and election. For if you do these things, you will never stumble,

2 Peter 1:10

Discover your spiritual gifts.

Take an online test to discover top 5 strengths at https://high5test.com.

Or

Print and take a paper test at SpiritualGiftsTest.com at https://spiritualgiftstest.com/wp-content/uploads/2019/03/adult-gifts-test.pdf

Or

Take a survey that your church uses.

These surveys only provide an indication of your spiritual gifts. Other ways to discover your gifts, talents, and purpose are

Serve in various capacities in your church and community. List areas to serve.

_____

_____

_____

1. Answer these questions as you expand your horizons.
    a. What gives you joy?

_____

_____

_____

    b. Where are you bearing fruit?

_____

_____

_____

    c. What do other people say about your work/ministry?

_____

_____

_____

2. Take action. Do not just sit around waiting for God. He will reveal your unique purpose as you act on what He reveals to you.

_____

_____

_____

   a. Read 2 Timothy 1:6. Write down action steps that will stir up your gift. Allow God to direct you.

_____

_____

_____

_____

   b. Read James 1:5. Ask God for Wisdom.

_____

_____

_____

c. Read James 4:2. Ask God for direction and revelation. Tell Him you want to do what He has created and called you to do.

_____

_____

_____

_____

_____

3. What direction is God sending you? Your purpose is unique, not like anyone else's. You have a niche that only you can nurture and fulfill. Once you know from God, then don't allow anyone else to control or direct the course of your life except God. Describe God's direction. Why do you believe it is from God?

_____

_____

_____

_____

_____

4. Write about what God is revealing to you. What is your calling? What is your purpose. What do you do different from anyone else?

_____

_____

_____

_____

_____

_____

_____

_____

_____

_____

_____

_____

24: The Church's Calling

But you are a chosen people, a royal priesthood, a holy nation, God's special possession, that you may declare the praises of him who called you out of darkness into his wonderful light.

1 Peter 2:9

We know that God is calling the church to be welcoming and inclusive. Where is your church or organization in the process?

_____

_____

_____

_____

_____

_____

_____

Find a local church that is inclusive of people with disabilities. Joni & Friends is a good source.

Email webpage: https://www.joniandfriends.org/about/contact-us/

Call or Text: 818-707-5664

Remember that a fully inclusive church takes work and time. Churches that have committed to people with disabilities are in various stages of the process.

Church Name:

_____

Address:

_____

_____

Phone:

_____

Contact person:

_____

Observations:

_____

_____

_____

_____

_____

_____

_____

_____

_____

_____

_____

_____

_____

Now, look around at your church.

Is your church going through a transition? Has there recently been an influx of people with disabilities? How is the church handling the change?

_____

_____

_____

_____

Do people with disabilities visit once or twice and never come again?

_____

_____

_____

Are there people or families affected by disability that attend on Sunday but are not involved with church activities? Describe.

_____

_____

_____

_____

What assistance has been provided for people with disabilities? Are there some people who needed more assistance than was provided?

_____

_____

_____

_____

_____

Where is your church in the transition process? Is your church planning for a future that includes people with disabilities? Why or Why not?

_____

_____

_____

_____

_____

_____

_____

_____

_____

What can you do to help? Be practical and creative with your resources
and time.

_____

_____

_____

_____

_____

_____

_____

_____

_____

_____

_____

_____

Conclusion

We realize that people with disabilities are part of God's plan for His church. As we foster an atmosphere of love and respect, we demonstrate our willingness to learn and grow as the body of Christ.

As you implement the strategies outlined, I pray you will be enlightened and excited. As we invite and bring people with disabilities to the banquet, our table will be full. As each part of the body functions properly, we can move together to advance the Kingdom of God.

Inclusion Education

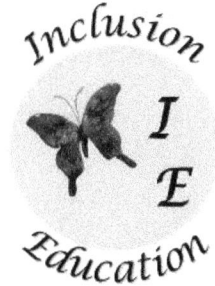

Toward Full Inclusion of People with Disabilities

Areas of Expertise	**Training Arenas**
Disability Sensitivity	Training Materials
Disability Etiquette	Consultations
Disability Ministry	Workshops
Accommodations	Seminars

Contact Information

Inclusion Education

727-945-2299

(Call or Text)

Debbie.Malone@inclusioneducation.com

www.inclusioneducation.com

FaceBook.com/DebbieMalone510

Additional Services: Ghostwriting: memoirs, faith-based books, web content

Individualized Solutions for Accessibility and Inclusion

DEBBIE MALONE

www.ingramcontent.com/pod-product-compliance
Lightning Source LLC
Chambersburg PA
CBHW051345290326
41933CB00042B/3184